Pocket

Holistic Healing

Dr. Ilona Melman

Astrolog Publishing House

Pocket Healing Books

Holistic Healing
Dr. Ilona Melman

Aromatherapy
Kevin Hudson

Reiki
Chantal Dupont

Vitamins
Jon Tillman

Introduction

Healing is a form of natural medicine whose operating principle is loving touch instead of medications.

Healing is the expression of a natural human propertyzand most accessible form of healing for everyone.

Everything in the universe consists of energy and is expressed through it. When a person touches an object - plant or animal - gently and lovingly, he transmits his energy to it in a natural way. When the person's body is in a normal, healthy condition, it balances itself, but a deviation from the normal condition leads to illness, and this is when the healing touch of the healer is required. The healer creates an environment of healing, balance and health, by means of which the patient's balance can be restored. The healer lays his hands on the patient's body, or holds them near to it, radiates energies of warmth and light through them, and the patient responds. While every person is a natural healer, there are people with stronger healing powers, either innate or acquired. The healer becomes a kind of intermediary who enables the energy level in the patient's body to become healthy.

Ilona Melman, Ph.D

1. Healing as a holistic treatment

If we hone our awareness, we will realize that there is a direct connection between our physical body and our feelings and thoughts. Our awareness of our health begins the moment we focus our attention on the fact that if we get angry or upset, we also suffer from headaches, nausea, muscle pains, or other symptoms; and if we are contented and happy, our body is healthier and more vital. There is often a link between our inability to release ourselves and be spontaneous on the one hand, and constipation on the other, or between shouldering burdens and responsibility on the one hand, and painful, hunched shoulders on the other.

When this topic was examined scientifically, it transpired that changes in thought and emotion produce biochemical changes in the brain. Mental tension manifests itself in moodiness, in disturbing thoughts, and in backaches. In these situations, electrical changes in the skin can be checked. In a state of tension, our muscles contract, affecting our blood circulation and the functioning of our glands and nerves; as a result, our entire body seizes up. This may well affect digestion, and lead to constipation. In order to deal with the problem, we may take a laxative. This is how we treat the symptoms, but not the root of the problem that is causing us to be constipated. On the other hand, holistic healing treats the entire person: body, mind and spirit (thought). Healing is a holistic - whole - cure, whose aim is to reach the source of the illness.

According to the quantum theory, everything in the universe vibrates with energy. Every person is an individuum, which means undivided, whole. A physical ailment can be produced by an unhealthy emotion or thought. Healing is a method of diagnosing the source of the disease and treating it using a holistic approach. During a healing treatment, the healer radiates healing energy onto the patient. In this way, the healing touch of the healer helps the patient experience feelings of release, balance, serenity, and joy in every sense: body, mind, and soul.

Researchers of healing have noticed the fact that when a person who is full of vitality, joy, serenity, and love is in the presence of a person who is ill or lacking in vitality, and especially when there is physical contact between them, a kind of energy exchange occurs (similar to the law of connected vessels). In principle, it is not possible for one person to heal another person, because only the person can heal himself (just like our skin can heal itself after an injury by natural cell regeneration), but the healer helps by creating a suitable recovery environment, which produces the required balance for the patient's body to heal itself. The healer creates the appropriate circumstances for healing, but the inner freedom to choose to receive vital energy and allow it to penetrate and renew the body lies with the patient.

The patient's body absorbs energy from the healer, and distributes it throughout the body. Then a scientifically proved biochemical change occurs: glands resume functioning, enzymes start working again, the nerves calm down, and blood circulation improves. All this has an emotional effect on the patient, who feels release, relief, joy, and happiness. This energy is considered to be magnetic. The patient-recipient's energy is attracted like a magnet to the healer's energy, similar to the connection between a mother and her sick child. A healer who has an abundance of vital energy is naturally a better magnetic healer, and many patients can renew their strength and be healed by him, by being beside him or by means of the touch of his hand. Having said this, the healer must safeguard his energy all the time, and renew it, so that it does not decrease. Healing that is performed correctly will prevent such a decrease.

When the healer allows this energy to flow through him, he links up to universal energy, and channels it (like an agent or intermediary) to the patient who is lacking in it. This is the healing action in the spiritual dimension. A professional and mature healer is gifted with a sense that enables him to absorb the type of universal energy that matches the electric vibrations in the patient's body. This sense, whose source is apparently in the pineal gland on the posterior side of the brain, is more developed and open in healers than in other people. The manner in which this gland opens, as well as the extent of its activity and power, provide the healer with his healing powers. The healer is likely to penetrate into the patient's hidden inner strata, affording a diagnosis of his problems, and the recovery of his way of thinking. This kind of diagnosic healing is called spiritual healing, and it requires that the healer develop his power of mind.

Wholeness and balance in the body, mind and soul

The concept of "disease" is easier to define than that of "health." The word "disease" means "dis-ease" - a temporary feeling of discomfort. According to the homeostatic theory of the psychologist, V. Cannon (1920), our body is equipped with a supply of medications, and we have natural rehabilitation and balance mechanisms. For instance, when our body is burning with fever, it tries to expel the fever by means of perspiration; or after an injury, there is cell regeneration. However, even a slight lack of harmony or balance in the body or mind suffices for the person to contract a disease. According to researcher V. Oldfield, every cell in the body vibrates at a particular and unique frequency that is controlled by the brain. In Oldfield's opinion, disease occurs because of a change in the body's electro-magnetic waves, causing a change in the normal flow of energy. In this way, the rhythm or vibration of the cells and organs changes to the point of deviating from equilibrium. If this situation continues chronically, it will lead to disease. A person who is aware, and who develops the ability to heed the inner early-warning signals, is sensitive to the moment he becomes weak, and can stop the disease before it worsens.

Health is defined as wholeness and balance in the body, mind, and spirit:

The health of our physical body depends on nutrition (minerals, vitamins) that is exactly suited to our needs, as well as rest, liquids, exercise, clean air, and ecology; it also depends on heredity and environment. The more we heed the early-warning signals about our health, the better.

Our emotional body is healthy if we are not blocked by anger, fears, hatred, grudges, sadness, jealousy, and so on, or trapped by unreleased emotions such as those mentioned above. In other words, emotions change the biochemical-enzymatic reactions in the body, and are liable to harm the immune system, just like every state of stress does. It is a good idea to prevent this by means of treatments such as breathing, yoga, meditation and relaxation, consciousness-raising treatments, and so on.

The spiritual-mental body - the thinking part - affects the rest of the systems by means of the central (cerebral) nervous system. Every thought is a form of energy with a structure or electro-magnetic field, which can exert an effect on disease or on health. In this way, too, memories of things past that are stored in the brain radiate their influence. Thoughts reflecting depression, worry, guilt, and so on, alter the biochemical state of the brain, and have a physiological effect.

2. The aim of healing

The aim of healing is to balance the life energy of the patient, and get it to flow along different paths. Healing is a journey of self-discovery. Because of various injuries in our past, and in order to survive, we developed a kind of protective armor around our energy field, which prevented us from experiencing unpleasant emotions - and then we became ill. The diagnosis and cure of the disease are an expression of the same self-discovery.

In the same way as the body can suffer from exhaustion as a result of a lack of vitamins and minerals in our food, or a lack of physical exercise, it can express a change in our vital state as a result of various tension blockages. According to experience and photographs, vital energy is liable to become weak. For example, a person who has difficulty responding, who represses anger, and who swallows insults over a long period of time, is eventually liable to become ill, according to the energetic theory of healing, with recurring sore throats, hoarseness, laryngitis, and so on. A closed person who does not vent his feelings ("eats himself up inside") is likely to develop an ulcer. The healer diagnoses the source of the illness and activates his healing energy. While touching the throat or abdominal area of the patients in the above examples, it is highly probably that the healer will experience feelings such as heat, prickling, heaviness, and so on, which stem from the blocked or shrunken energy.

Sometimes, the source of the disease is found at a distance from the place in which the symptom is manifested. For instance, when the person complains of migraines, the source of the problem may be in the region of the heart (this attests to confusion or frustration), or in the lower back region (this attests to a feeling of a lack of support). The moment the healer identifies the source of the problem, he musters his healing powers, and by uniting his energies with those of the patient, a healing electrical field is created. After a period of healing (sometimes several treatments), it is almost certain that the balance of the patient's powers will be restored.

3. The healer

Qualities of the healer

Unconditional love: The dominant quality that is a prerequisite for a healing practitioner is unconditional love. The healer acquires this quality during the course of his spiritual development. Other qualities, such as devotion, love that derives from compassion and does not expect anything in return, preparation, the desire to help, give, and dedicate himself unselfishly, modesty, listening, sensitivity to others and to himself, altruism, faith in himself and in others - all increase with time, experience, and spiritual development. Tools such as meditation, inner scrutiny and listening, and especially the faith and the will to heal, are likely to help.

Unity - integration: At the height of a healing treatment, the healer operates from coordinated brain waves. From research conducted on healers' brains during healing treatments, it transpired that in most of them, there was a perfect correlation between brain wave patterns on the left and right sides, which work at a certain rhythm similar to the frequency of the magnetic field of the earth (Shuman waves). These results were verified in similar research that was conducted by Maxwell Kidd and Geoff Blendel, who found that this state of brain waves in the pattern of matching alpha waves on the two sides of the brain is similar to the state of deep rest or relaxation. This is analogous to the example of wholeness-unity or inner integration, in which the healer is at the height of the act of healing, and it is possible that this is the reason why he succeeds at healing.

Mediation: The healer serves as a kind of pipeline for transferring universal life force with a "high field" of energy between himself and the patient, whose energy state is not as good. The patient musters the energy necessary for his recovery via the healer.

The healer's training

Both healers who were born with an exceptional ability to heal, and others who were born with lesser powers, can progress by developing these powers. Centers for studying healing exist all over the world. The bulk of the healer's development occurs along his own spiritual path: by experience through trial and error. Because of the individual nature of healing, it is difficult to formulate it in terms of empirical research. Today, in any case, there is documentation of results based on the experience that has accumulated up until now.

4. The healing force as life force

The healing force is an expression of the life energy or the universal energy field. The human aura is an expression of this power. Researchers in various cultures have tried to investigate the healing force. The following table presents a historical survey of these investigations (according to the research of B. Brennan).

Year	*Researcher/Place*	*Name of Energy*
5000 BC	**India**	**Prana**

The finding: The basic life source; it is expressed in breathing.

3500 BC	**Egypt**	**Supernatural powers**

The finding: Exist in special places in nature.

3000 BC	**China**	**Chi, Yin and Yang**

The finding: Energy exists in everything. Yin and yang are polar forces; when they are balanced, the person becomes healthy.

500 BC	**Pythagoras / Greece**	**Vital energy**

The finding: Healing forces vs. harmful forces, illuminating bodies that engender healing.

1200 AD	**Paracelsus / Europe**	**Aliaster**

The finding: Vital force for healing. Spiritual, energetic work, invisible "steam," "magnet," "vapor" that envelops a warm body. A change in the composition of the magnetic vapor causes sickness or health. There are people who influence the sheath of magnetic energy of sick people by transmitting radiation through their fingertips.

1800 AD	**Dr. Anton Mesmer / France, Vienna**	**Magnetic field**

The finding: Can charge inanimate and animate objects, hypnotism, influence from a distance. That is, there is an energetic-magnetic force that influences living things without the need for physical contact or chemical interference. Tried by him first with magnetic rods, water, and hypnotism. Attempted successfully to transmit healing from healer to patient.

1800 AD	**W. von Leibniz**	**Essential element**

The finding: Centers of forces that contain their own *motion engines*.

1800 AD	**G. von Reichenbach**	**Fire power**

The finding: Compares to an electro-magnetic field.

1902-1910		**Whirlpool of energy**

The finding: The connection to the chakras - energy centers in the framework of theosophical studies.

1911	**W. Kilner**	**Aura - human atmosphere**

The finding: Used a colored screen to see three layers in the aura, diagnosis of the disease according to the layers of the aura.

1930-1940	**S. Kirlian**	**Aura photography**

The finding: For the first time, the features of the aura were photographed. An ethereal layer as a manifestation of electric discharge, an electro-magnetic field that reflects health or blockages in energy flow.

1940	**G. de la Ware**	**Flowing and radiation**

The finding: Invention of "radionic" tools for discovering radiation from live tissues for diagnosis and distance healing.

1930-1950 W. Reich Orgone

The finding: The discovery of a form of psychotherapy that applies the energy of orgone in the human body. Investigated the energy in nature, and ways to collect the orgone.

1930-1960 R. Borph. Northrop Life force

The finding: Life force builds a structure of organisms and develops ideas of the rhythm of cycles.

1950 L. Rawitz Thought field

The finding: Thought field with life force for creating psychosomatic symptoms.

1970-1989 R. Becker Electro-magnetic field

The finding: A measure for an electro-magnetic field that is changeable, and that changes physical and psychological manifestations. Discovered a method for controlling systematic currents in the human body in conjunction with illness and health. Discovered an approach that contains self-growth of the electric current. The tensions are organized in representative electric fields similar to the meridians and the nervous system.

1970-1980 Brennan High "super powers"

The finding: Correlation of clinical energetic field in coordination with emotional reaction.

1970-1990 R. Motoyama Chi

The finding: An electrical index and meridians (energy currents) in acupuncture served to diagnose and treat illnesses. The tensions are organized in electrical fields that represent power lines intersecting the meridians, mainly at acupuncture points or at ganglia (nerve intersections), or energy bodies that are connected to the ethereal body (the body that is close to the physical body in the aura).

1970-1980 **Bioplasma**

The finding: Life force as bioplasma composed of free ions. All the states of positive/negative ions determine health.

1970-1980 **V. Hunt** **Biofield**

The finding: Electrical index for frequencies and the location of the meta-biofield in humans, in coordination with aura readers and interpreters.

1960-1990 **A.P. Herritz** **The field that defines life**

The finding: Magnetic force was measured from healers' hands, and were found to be about 7-8 Hertz. Higher or lower occurrence than this determines "life."

1980-1990 **R. Beck** **Shuman wavés**

The finding: Compares magnetic beats in coordination with the rhythm of the magnetic field of the earth.

1980-1990 **G. Zimmerman** **Brain waves**

The finding: Shows that the brain waves of the healer turn to left/right matching (synchronization) of "alpha" brain waves in accordance with what happens to the patient as well.

1990-1993 **Dr. V. Miller** **Para electricity and wholeness**

The finding: "The vital energy" of every person is identical to Chi, to Prana (Chinese Yoga), to fire power, to orgone, to "field of life" (of Bohr), and so on.

5. Scientific examination of the influence of healing

The influence of healing on plants: Plants constitute a measure for discovering the results of energetic healing. From healing treatments performed on plants, it transpires that their growth rate increased for a long time.

The influence of healing on water: Healing energy that was radiated by a healer on water changed its properties. The healing treatment caused a change (decrease) in the water's surface tension, and in another case in its hydrogen links and its electrical properties (similar to the changes following treatment with a magnet).

Water that underwent healing treatment changed the color of the solution of copper chloride crystals that crystallize in a salt solution. This constitutes a possible measure for the presence of healing energy and the possibility of measuring it.

The influence of healing on enzymatic activity: The researcher, Dr. Smith, conducted research in which she discovered how healing forces influence enzymes (digestion catalysts). She examined the forces of a healer called K. Estebani, and gave him a certain enzyme for healing treatment. Her research revealed that the force or energy that flowed from the healer's hands activated the enzyme both quantitatively and qualitatively.

The influence of healing on the hemoglobin level in the blood: The research of M. Grad and B. Smith constituted the basis for Prof. Craiger's research in the USA. From her research on the life force ("Prana") in the air, it transpires that Prana is an inseparable part of the oxygen molecules in the air. In consequence, she examined the hemoglobin level in the blood (the carrier of oxygen in the blood) in patients before and after healing. She concluded that there was a change, and that their hemoglobin level had improved.

6. Types of healing

Healing by physical contact

After preparation and personal recharging, the healer uses his fingers to survey and diagnose the source of the disease or its cause. Afterward, he places his hands on the patient's body for a few minutes or more, as needed, until recovery occurs. The healer has several ways of intensifying his powers, just as a battery is recharged. He can use breathing, prayer, relaxation, concentration, visualization, colors, and so on to help him - until he unites with the force that is flowing from his head to his hands. The "purer" and "cleaner" his energy is, the stronger it is and the better the results of the treatment will be.

Distant healing

This kind of treatment, which is also called "absent healing," is performed when the healer sends the healing to a patient who is far from him - even many kilometers away. This is done by means of directing the healer's thinking in a mental and visualizing way.

The aim of this treatment is to send treatment to people who feel bad and are not mobile or have no way of getting to a healer. Healing energy is universal, is found everywhere, and is not limited by time, distance or place. According to this theory, energy flows along the thought path, so that it is possible to concentrate and channel it in different ways: by concentrating on a photograph of the patient, or by visualizing him; by using colors, crystals, or other means.

Group healing

In order to intensify the effect of the healing, it is possible to get a group of healers together, and obtain especially powerful results. Experience has shown that the effect of such a healing is infinitely greater than that of a single healer (an analogous situation would be a laser beam as opposed to the beam of a flashlight). The entire group focuses together, either imagining or in physical contact with the afflicted organ of the patient. It turns out that the strength of the combined treatment is greater than that of the individual treatments, and the improvement is shown to be faster.

Self-healing

It is a good idea to learn self-healing. In that way, the patient can take responsibility for his treatment and intensify it. The "Reiki Healing" method is also highly recommended as a method of recharging for the healer himself, and therefore self-healing is learned and developed. In this method, all the energy centers in the body are purified every day, thus allowing a better flow and charge of energy, and improving it, so as to prevent disease as well.

7. Methods of healing

Bio-energy

The bio-energy method was developed by the psychologist W. Reich in the 1930s. By means of various experiments, Reich discovered energy that he called "orgone," and identified unique properties in it. An energy field or life force, "orgone," is found in the body and outside it, in every living, growing, or inanimate substance, in humans, in the atmosphere, in the sky, and in every empty space. This is the life energy that penetrates every place in various forms and densities. It expands and contracts, flows from a more concentrated place to a less concentrated place, and vice versa. This energy affects organisms at a distance. It is influenced by sounds, and can be controlled by consciousness. It flows along thought paths, can be stored in various vessels such as boxes or cans, can be measured quantitatively, and linked to water and magnets.

According to this method, the energy field ("orgone") of every living creature, from an ameba to a human being, that is injured (for instance, pricked by a pin, beaten up, or feels fear or anger), will contract in the injured place and will never forget it. At the time, the contraction acted as a defense and survival mechanism, but later on the place became hard and "armored," and may have formed a kind of "lump," "growth," or "heat," that needed a lot of unnecessary energy to preserve it, and then the organism gets ill. This state is called "blockage," and the healer works on this energy field using the method of bio-energy.

First he has to find out which hand absorbs energy from the body and releases blockages, and which hand gives healing energy. In this treatment, there are different forms of contact besides gentle and mainly strong massage, energy draining, various ways of breathing, and treatment accessories (orgone machine, various blankets, etc.).

Magnetic healing

Anton Mesmer was a physician who investigated hypnosis and its action at the end of the 18th and the beginning of the 19th centuries. He believed that there was a force of magnetic energy that could affect living beings without the necessity for physical contact or chemical intervention. In other words, by means of transmitting or charging magnetic energy, it is possible to cure people whose energetic system is injured. He began to treat patients with magnetic rods, water and hypnosis, in order to transmit energy from the healer to the patient and cure him. He opened clinics in Vienna and Paris, and his success rate in curing diseases was extremely high in comparison to conventional medicine. Mesmer first used rods and magnets, but later reached the conclusion that this energy could be transmitted most effectively directly from the healer to the patient via the palms. Despite his success, Mesmer was deported from France, and his method was shelved for many years. However, his influence in using hypnosis and in curing by healing was enormous.

Empirical scientific research examined the use and effect of the magnet in healing and curing:

In a photograph, a strong electro-magnet can be seen sending its "field" right through the flesh, blood and bones of the hand, and "arranging" iron filings. This force is even stronger than the force of gravity, and holds the filings exactly along the "force lines" of the magnetic field. (This makes it easier to understand that similar "fields," which surround every living and inanimate substance, organize it in unique shapes and preserve the shapes.)

In a special photograph of the fields of the aura (see Chapter 9: The aura), the magnetized steel needle of a compass was photographed, with its lower end shifting the energy field of a leaf. This experiment indicates the effect of the magnet on the leaf's aura field.

A magnet and healing on the electro-magnetic field change the molecular structure of water and of other substances.

From experience, it transpires that there is a connection between the location of the healer and the results of the healing. A healer by the name of B. Harris discovered that she sharpened her healing force and her sight if she sat with her back toward the north pole.

Bioplasmic healing

This healing was first introduced by Soviet scientists. In parallel to the term "ethereal," the term "bioplasmic" relates to the tendency to consider it a fourth state of matter (that is, plasma alongside solid, liquid, and gas). It seems that the bioplasmic body does not use electrical energy as a material body, but another vital energy. It now seems, according to this healing theory, that via centers of hidden energy, called "chakras," and via the flow of "meridians" and acupuncture points, the body receives partially magnetic energy (similar to the expression "para-electrical energy field," according to Warhol). According to this, the chakras are invisible whirlpools of energy that channel non-material energy to the internal secretory glands, and from them by means of the inner energy lines.

During healing, energy exchanges occur between the chakra systems of the healer and the patient. This healing is based on the writings of the theosophist A. Bailey, who saw the basis for it in the ethereal (plasmatic) source. She claimed that it was a ubiquitous life force that preceded energy, and in the human body, there are lines and ints in which this force exists and flows. This flow is also called "meridians," according to Oriental philosophy.

In parallel to the flow of blood in the veins, arteries, and capillaries, which gives vitality to every form of life, there is another body, called the "astral" body (the body of emotion), and the source of most diseases is found in both strata - the ethereal and the astral - especially psychosomatic diseases that reveal no pathological findings in laboratory tests. It is possible to find the source of these diseases and to treat them by means of the bioplasmic energy approach.

The whole approach is based on the writings of *Chang Chai* from the 11th century (1020) and the Oriental philosophical writings, vedas, and spiritual writings, in which it is written that the "ethereal," like the Chi, forms the shapes of all things, actions and organs. The anthroposophist, R. Steiner (from Bailey's time) called it "the creative forces," in which he saw the molds for every level of life.

Religious and secular spiritual healing

Spiritual healing is performed by means of transferring thoughts by telepathy, and demands high-level spiritual forces. Russian scientists who conducted a series of experiments during the last decade (1980-1990) clearly proved that one person is capable of influencing the thoughts and physiological reactions of another person, even at a distance of thousands of kilometers. It is not yet understood what the nature of this energy is, and at what level it is transferred (by means of the pineal gland in the brain, or in the subconscious via the chakras, or in another way), but according to the results of such a healing, its existence has not been denied. In this method, the healer focuses his inner being, his breathing, or his spirit, very deeply, and is capable of healing the injured organ or the patient "in his imagination" until recovery is effected. This treatment can be helped by the patient's objects - a photograph, for example - by means of which the healer transmits his healing force.

Another finding shows that during meditation, the eyes transmit a lot of energy. This can be seen in thermographic photos, which are photos of heat emission from objects. During the treatment, an increased heat emission was found in the region of the eyes. The same is true for the healer's voice. This research, which was conducted in the USA, in England, and in Russia, also reveals telekinesis (moving objects). From here, it was proved that the concentration of the healer's consciousness is likely to bring about molecular and biochemical changes, as well as healing the body. According to the research of Dr. Elmer Green and Jack Schwartz in 1972, which was presented in a lecture at Stanford University in the USA, it transpires that it is possible to stop bleeding by means of the power of thought, and control infections in the body by means of contact between the healer and the patient. Furthermore, it is possible to influence the growth rate of plants, or increase the rate of production of red blood cells in the patient, leading to his recovery. This process requires caution, responsibility, seriousness, and the *patient's* permission, and it must be done under careful supervision.

Spiritual healing also exists in the religious realm. Prayer and blessing constitute a type of healing. From ancient times until today, prayer and blessing comprise a strong, suggestive healing force in various cultures and religions. The sound, the melody, the word, and the vibrations that they produce help healing. By means of symbols (such as the Star of David or the crucifix) and other objects (crystals), and especially by means of intention (and direction), when the healer communicates his request for help in his prayer to the "superior force" in order to do something for others who need help - the person who is blessing becomes a kind of emissary or intermediary between the superior forces and the patient. In the Jewish, Christian, or any other religion, there are spiritual healers who use holy places as a place for healing, for example, a church or the graves of saints. Spiritual leaders draw spiritual strength from the place itself. Prayer operates as a force of inspiration. Prayer with intention constitutes a kind of energetic template, which helps recovery and healing.

Mental healing

Mental healing is performed by means of visualizing the patient as a person who is recovering (or is already healthy), or when the patient is in a state in which his brain is radiating alpha waves, or he is hearing alpha sound with movements and touches on his hands.

The Silva method: In the Silva Mind Control method, healing and development can be achieved through the reduction of tension, by controlling the brain so that it operates on low frequencies, close to the frequency of alpha waves.

The known frequencies of brain waves are:

Beta frequency (14-21 cycles per second): during thinking, consciousness, daydreaming.

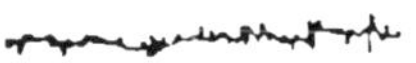

Alpha frequency (7-14 cycles per second): during relaxation, meditation, before falling asleep or before daydreaming.

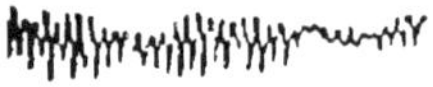

Theta frequency (4 cycles per second): during sleep.

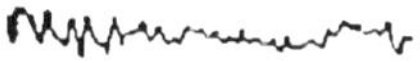

Delta frequency (fewer than 4 cycles per second): during deep sleep, under anesthesia.

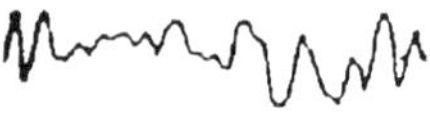

The patient listens to alpha sound (on a frequency of 7-14 cycles per second), imagines his sick body becoming healthy, and sees this occurring clearly in his imagination. In this way, the patient can supervise his health.

José Silva was an electronics technician by profession. During the course of his research, he discovered that the electrical functioning of the brain, reaching the point of creating alpha waves, constituted a way of logging on to inner healing. This is similar to the state of relaxation, and, as has already been mentioned, it is possible to achieve the best healing results both singly and in healing groups.

The superology method: Another method of mental healing is the superology method. According to the founder of the method, Dr. Alphonse Caissado, there is a state between wakefulness and sleep (the superological state (in which the brain also transmits alpha waves).

With this method, people learn to relax muscles, to concentrate on the body (on the pulse, temperature, breathing, and so on), and see the future state of serenity they yearn for. This method consists of yoga techniques and meditative seeing and listening exercises, and aims to cure body and soul.

Biofeedback is an interim method between the two above mentioned methods, and it too helps in self-healing. According to this approach, it is possible to get into an alpha state by means of a biofeedback instrument, which emits signals every time the person reaches the desired state of relaxation. In this method, the person can recover from various diseases, tensions, hypertension, headaches, and many other syndromes, and he learns to control the tensions and pressures that caused the disease.

Psychocybernetics: According to this theory, the brain operates like a computer and a control system. By means of mental thinking, and mainly through guided imagining, it is possible to cure diseases. The originators of the method, Emile Coúe, Maltz, and others, developed a way in which it is possible to change the condition of the immune system by means of thought and its direction via suggestion. (For instance, we can help heal a cut in the body by imagining cells growing and knitting the injured region together, or we can improve the functioning of the immune system if we imagine white blood cells reproducing and succeeding in fighting infections and malignant tumors.) Since thought power has an extremely high level of healing energy, it is possible to recover from diseases (even terminal ones) in the best possible way with this method. Suggestion in this method (just like in other visualization methods) operates on the endless repetition of positive thoughts and affirmations that link up with the subconscious. It is possible to recover from and cure every disease by mustering the inner healing forces in this way.

Healing with love

Healing is love, and therefore an obstacle in love's path causes disease and imbalance. There is a connection between love and reinforcement and the immune glands in the body, and that is why healing depends on it. The healing methods of Dr. K. Simenton and Dr. B. Segal advocate certain elements, at the head of which is love as the greatest healing force. Love is the true miracle that can cancel or apply the laws of nature, especially if it comes from the heart, from the soul, and unconditionally. When it flows, it affords a feeling of unity and wholeness, purifies energies, and produces the highest possibility for healing. Self-love is the heart of healing, and at the next stage, it can be transmitted to others.

Dr. Simenton, who was one of the pioneers in oncology and cancer-curing in the USA, discovered that by effecting a basic change in beliefs, by means of self-love and repeated "guided imagining," it is possible to alter the condition of a patient (even of terminal cancer patients). Within 3-6 weeks, if the treatment is repeated consistently several times a day, an improvement in the state of health can be achieved. According to his cumulative research and experiments, Dr. Simenton reckoned that prolonged tension destroyed the natural ability of the cells in our body to defend and cure themselves. If the body is given the opportunity, it will heal itself. Both Dr. Simenton and Dr. Segal, author of the book, "Love, Medicine and Miracles," advocate this healing method, especially for cancer patients. In this method, the basic beliefs that led to the disease are changed by means of the suggested exercises; many people recovered as a result of the method, with the help of faith and a great deal of love.

Healing with vibrations (frequencies)

Radiesthesia (pendulum): This is a method of diagnosis, treatment and distant healing whose aim is to locate the exact cause of the disease and find the appropriate treatment for it. According to this approach, every cell and organ in the body vibrates at its own particular rhythm. Deviation from the rhythm or from the connection to other rhythms as wholeness causes imbalance and consequently disease. The healer makes contact with the patient by means of some of his hair, a picture of him, a nail paring, or other objects, and uses a pendulum that acts as an intermediary between the conscious and the subconscious, the intuition, the healing force, and the knowledge of the healer. In this way, the healer can ascertain whether the cause of the disease lies in the person's physical, emotional, or spiritual body, and in which organ the balance has been disrupted. This is a holistic approach, in which healing is performed by means of vibrations of the currents of electro-magnetic energy, through which diagnosis and healing are effected. The pendulum is a radionic instrument that operates as a monitor which is sensitive to the ethereal realm, that is, it absorbs the patient's energy. Its function is to focus the external energy and send it into the person's aura sheath after the cause of the disease has been identified (not just in the physical body). In addition, the pendulum serves as a delicate and sensitive seismograph (alongside the rest of the routine tests). This method is not simply diagnostic, but rather also therapeutic and balancing, and it restores the rhythm of the organs' vibration to normal.

Healing with crystals: R. Oldfield, one of the researchers of aura photography, claims that every cell in our body vibrates at a rate that is determined and controlled by the brain, and that diseases are caused by a change in the electro-magnetic waves of the body and by an impaired energy flow. In order to rectify this situation, it is possible to use the electro-magnetic field of crystals, especially of quartz crystals, that form and change the energy field, and thus help cure diseases. Another researcher, A. Harold, recommends using crystals for healing plants and animals, for balancing energy centers, and for relaxation, thus bringing about general healing.

Quartz crystals have a geometric structure that matches the electro-magnetic field of the earth in a natural manner, and the energy received from this field stimulates the aura field of human beings. Electric energy is liberated from inside quartz crystals. This energy has a high and exact vibration, and in this way, it is possible to change the body's vibrational frequency for purposes of healing. When a negative emotion, such as anger or fear, affects the glands that are linked to the nervous system and the energy centers, causing blockages and illness, they can be "cleaned energetically" by means of crystals. Ailments such as migraine, hypertension, sores, broken bones, and so on, can be cured effectively with crystals, which reveal a kind of dimension that links the inanimate with the animate, especially when the crystal is clean, and then its flow is sharper. The crystal directs negative energy away from the patient, and cleans it. It can work on all the energy levels: body, mind, and spirit, and therefore it is holistic.

It is also an extremely powerful analytical tool, called a quartz generator. Mainly, it is possible to "transmit" the energy of "love" and "positive thoughts" to a crystal, and enhance healing. Since it is a kind of powerful transmitter for increasing the energy and a sort of magnetic battery, it spreads and radiates it powerfully. Crystals can be placed on the body itself, next to the body in a particular order, on the energy centers, or in a glass of water. The water is drunk (crystal extraction) or used to cleanse the body, the room, or any other place of negative energies.

Healing with sounds: Healing can be enhanced by sound or voice. The world was created by sound: "And God said: Let there be light." In order to become healthy, something must be created, and anything that disturbs the creature must be cured. The emission of sounds during healing is accepted practice with spiritual healers. During the healing session, they emit special sounds that create a vibration, and therefore a resonance is created in correlation with the cells and the organs in the body. David played to King Saul when he was deeply troubled, and he got well. Sound consists of vibrations that create shapes. In a laboratory experiment, a correlation was found between emitting sound and the creation of a shape. And so sounds can bring about a morphological, mental, emotion, and spiritual change, and can cure.

Thus, sounds and their special shape release and develop awareness, and heal. They change the rate of breathing and blood circulation, and they are the expression of hormonal secretion. Various healers use their voices (sometimes in a group) with the different vowels, such as *ah*, *eh*, *ee*, *oo* or *au*, which express the sounds of the energy centers (chakras), and heal by balancing them. There is a link between music and color, because both of them vibrate at frequencies that are interrelated. The emotional, spiritual (astral) world is affected by emotional vibrations such as music and color, and negative feelings can be channeled and transformed into an exuberant mood. When a person expresses himself in sound or color, and is affected by them, he is immersed (without being aware of it) in a meditative-like state, operates his right brain, and broadcasts "alpha waves." This is how he receives inspiration, and healing occurs.

Healing with color (chromotherapy): In ancient cultures in the Far East - China, India and Tibet, as well as the Near East - Egypt and Greece, color was used for healing. Over the years, the subject was perfected and studied scientifically and experientially by the Greeks, the Romans, Paracelsus, Goethe, and others. Color is the expression of a wave length, of a frequency, of a vibration, that matches the frequency of the cells, the organs, and the energetic system of the human body (as well as of every living plant and animal organism).

Our aura is an expression of color, and through it, the colors are expressed and transmitted to the energy centers (chakras). This is why colors serve as medications for the body, as they vibrate in a rhythm that matches equilibrium. There are many methods for healing with color: "inhaling," "eating" or "drinking" color: drinking water that has been filtered with a colored screen, eating food of the required color, wearing clothing in the color that is suitable for healing, staying in a place where the appropriate color dominates (in the furnishings, in the surroundings), washing in a bath of colored water, looking at stained glass or colors, illuminating with colored lamps, imagining colors during visualization or meditation, using colored crystals, and so on.

According to color researcher Babbit, who tried to heal by means of color, and investigated the subject scientifically, it is possible to write down how each of the colors affects the person. He assumed that blue calmed and relaxed the blood and the nerves; that when the person had a cold, or was sad or withdrawn, red was the appropriate color, as it stimulates the heart and the blood, and renews energy. For problems in the stomach and digestive organs, yellow is suitable; for intestinal problems, green; for reproductive organs, pink; for respiratory organs, orange, which also affects the production of calcium.

According to the well-known color researcher, A. Casey, the color red is linked to blood diseases and increased sexual desire; orange - to respiratory-pulmonary problems, various glands, and muscle cramps, to self-confidence and energy; yellow is beneficial for digestive and nervous problems; green helps headaches, and balances the body and the soul; blue operates against inflammations, and helps cool and soothe the body; purple helps with sensory problems, for spiritual development, and for spiritual enlightenment.

Polarity therapy

The method of polarity therapy was developed by R Stone, and is based on electrical polarity. According to this method, the body has two poles, just like a battery: positive and negative. In the healing process, the healer helps in the potential electrical change in the body, a change that brings about equilibrium in the body. The healer does this through contact, massage, and healing in the regions in which the electrical-energetic system is impaired. He adds or takes away electricity, in this way balancing the energy. It is known that batteries accelerate the growth of seedlings, and the addition of electricity, or the inversion of the poles, helps healing in general.

Reiki

Rei is superior, divine, universal wisdom, supernatural knowledge. It is spiritual consciousness that comes from the universe: divine consciousness that is omniscient, understands each person perfectly, understands the reasons for all problems and difficulties, and knows what to do to overcome them. Enlightenment arrives directly from creation in the form of energy.

Ki is the life force that is parallel to Prana (in Sanskrit), to Mana (in Hawaiian), to Chi (in Chinese), to *Fire* Force, to Bioplasm, to Orgone (Reich). It is also used in other energies (Tai Chi, Chi Kong). There are 32 types of Chi in the universe. This life force is not physical, but it motivates every living creature, flows in us, and envelops us. A person whose Chi is blocked is ill, and susceptible to illness. At the moment of death, Chi leaves the person.

Reiki is a method of linking up to cosmic energy in order to transmit universal life energy, and in order to heal people. Its source in Japan was discovered by Dr. Usui.

This life energy is expressed in a spiritual way, and guides itself by means of its own wisdom. It is within the grasp of the Reiki practitioner, who undergoes special training.

In this healing method, the hands are placed on the body or held at a short distance from it. They are navigated and directed by the cosmic energy via the healer. The energy knows its way in the diagnosis and location of the reason and the healing of the problem. It is helped by symbols, by exact energy channels. By means of hand positions on the energy centers, it is possible to cure diseases. The aim of the treatment is to balance the energies in the body that caused the diseases, either by self-healing or by healing others.

The symbols that are used in healing are ideograms - drawing-like signs with particular meanings - in which there are seven energetic levels, and their meaning is the link from the universal to the earthy. Via the symbols, the healer can link up in his mind with the energy channels, to Chi, to gather it and transmit it to the patient, and to balance the patient's energy field.

Reiki energy arrives directly from the cosmos, goes toward the belly, which is the largest energy center in the body (around the navel), and from there travels to every part of the body that needs balancing.

Reiki consists of two types of energy: polar-vertical (Shiva) and horizontal (Sakti). The body takes the type and the quantity that it needs. Since it is energy that is aware, it knows where, when and how much the body needs (masculine, feminine, more, less). As a result, the simple method of laying hands on various places in the body, from the head down to the feet, is concentrated and intensive. It has been proved to be extremely effective.

8. The treatment procedure in healing

Reactions to the treatment

The patient's reactions to healing can occur during or after the treatment. The healer creates a stimulus for accelerating the recovery process, and improves the balance in the body, mind, and spirit. This procedure causes a reaction in the patient. Healing is likely to help the person cleanse himself of medications and of waste that accumulates in his body as a result of his unhealthy lifestyle.

As opposed to invasive treatments, such as medications and surgery, which are essentially masculine, healing is essentially a "feminine" technique, and it gets rid of waste and balances. Healing therapy is reminiscent of a river that is blocked by a rock, and as a result, its flow is disrupted. "Getting rid of the rock" is like to balance "the river's renewed flow."

There are people who experience various reactions during the treatment, such as thermal reactions (heat and cold), electrical reactions (prickling, pins and needles, a current), magnetic reactions (a kind of stickiness), or emotional reactions: crying, joy, release, fatigue, heaviness, anger, fear, jubilation, happiness, relief, a great deal of energy, or "crying" reactions of the body: a runny nose, excretions, tears, shivers, dizziness or various pains, or things they had experienced in the past and had ostensibly been cured of. These reactions occur because the nervous systems encodes and store painful memories that the body has difficulty coping with for any length of time. During the healing, there is an opportunity to purify them and get rid of them permanently. Any kind of emotional tension is liable to cause an accumulation of waste, which is the result of chemical reactions in the cells. A patient can feel heat, which allows the breakdown of calcium accumulations, acids, or waste in the blood. He may feel a change in heart rate and various currents. He may feel pain, but also release. His face becomes clear, his eyes open, he can feel serene and happy. Situations of stress have physical manifestations: perspiration, tension, nervousness, hypertension, inner tremors, hormonal reaction such as increased adrenaline secretion, digestive pressure, and so on. The healer's "electro-magnetic" power, which is directed at healing, is likely to get rid of these manifestations of stress from the layers of the aura, and cleanse the energy centers (chakras). From there, the influence passes to the nervous systems, to the organs, to the hormonal systems, and to every cell in the body. The healer should inform the patient about the healing procedure and the reactions that may occur during and after the treatment; the patient must consent to the treatment, which might be protracted.

Counter-indications

The concept "counter-indications" defines the people who cannot receive healing treatment. In order for the treatment to succeed, it is important to sift out people who are not open or prepared to receive healing as an approach to cure, or who oppose it.

In cases of early pregnancy (and especially after many miscarriages), or of a person who has been taking many medications for years - the healer must operate cautiously, professionally, and in an extremely controlled manner. Special attention must be given to terminal cancer patients, to people undergoing surgery or just after it, to people with pacemakers, and to especially difficult psychosomatic situations. It must be pointed out that experienced healers report significant relief and improvement even in situations such as the ones mentioned above.

Diagnosis in healing

In conventional medicine, diagnosis is assisted by blood tests, CT scans, X-rays, bone scans, and so on. In healing, diagnosis is performed by scanning the state and balance of energy in the body via the energy centers (chakras), as well as the state of the aura layers: blockages that are manifested mainly in contractions, in non-flow, in excess or lack, in heat or cold, and are perceived in the aura layers.

In the Reiki Healing method, the healer scans the body from a short distance or nearer with the help of his hand. The healer feels reactions such as heat, cold, a kind of stickiness, currents, tremor, pins and needles, prickling, and so on, and these provide him with signals about the places where there is an imbalance in the body that has to be treated.

According to the bio-energy method, the question of which hand performs the examination is important. Every "lump" indicates a blockage, which shows a contraction in the region. Touching a place like this is liable to hurt, since it dredges up a painful emotional or physical experience from the past. The blockage must be located, as it drains a lot of energy from the body, tiring it out to the point of exhaustion and causing various diseases.

The patient's willingness to be treated by healing can be determined by a light touch beside the energy center on his forehead. Signals from this region in comparison with other regions can provide a great deal of information. A diagnosis can also come from intuitive spiritual feelings, which the healer develops. In order to help make the diagnosis, the healer can check the colors of the aura and examine the state of energy in the body by means of crystals and a pendulum.

Diagnosis by pendulum is based on the hypothesis that it is possible to obtain additional information about the energies in our bodies according to the link between the left and right sides of the brain. The pendulum picks up thin, delicate, internal levels of energy that cannot be discovered in any other way. It permits information to be retrieved from the subconscious, and helps many healers diagnose blockages in the delicate bodies. Since it operates according to bio-electrical principles, every blockage is manifested in a certain form of movement of the pendulum. By means of a suitable code, it is possible, to discover blockages and diseases, and even use it for healing at a later stage. The pendulum's movements can be compared before and after the treatment.

Another way of diagnosing is to examine the pulse of the pendulum. The comparison of the pulse before and after healing enables the healer to understand the changes in the energy flow in the body.

The process of primary diagnosis of the patient includes an interview, in which regular informative details about the patient are examined: previous illnesses, familial diseases, longevity, medications, results of lab tests, and so on. A skilled healer can glean a lot from the patient's body language during the interview, and from the intuitive impression he receives from the patient. The healer requires the ability to listen as well as a great deal of experience in this field. In order to link up to the patient's real frequency, the healer uses his intuition and spiritual strength.

An important part of the diagnosis is the diagnosis of the colors of the aura. Every color is a frequency that stores important information about the energy of the entire person.

The healer's energetic protections

Since the healer is assisted by the ethereal energies that are especially delicate, and he is exposed to the patient's energetic waste, he can be harmed if he has not learned to empty himself. For this reason, the healer has to take measures to safeguard himself.

He must prepare the healing room in a way that suits his purpose, so that it constantly fills up with positive and healing energy. The room must be aired continuously, as negative energy tends to be compressed and to disrupt. The healer should breathe fresh air all the time, drink a lot of water before and after every treatment, and burn incense and essential oils (which purify the energetic atmosphere by spreading nourishing energies). The healer should not eat too much before the treatment, and he should wash his hands and, if possible, shower before and after treatments, thus purifying his aura.

It is also a good idea for the healer to engage in relaxation, meditation, prayer, and direction, so as to help other people with love and compassion, and to develop the concept of unconditional love. The room can be filled with healing stones - quartz and other crystals - in order to charge the room all the time. Especially recommended are crystals that are clear and sparkling after washing and purification. Plants, flowers, pleasing pictures, and relaxing music in the room all enhance the atmosphere, as does suitable, quiet clothing for the healer. He must make every effort to eliminate all noises, unpleasant odors, dirt, and untidiness. Before the treatment, the healer should imagine himself "enveloped in a pyramid of light" or in a "bubble of light" that protects him and provides him with energy for pure breathing - "Prana" breathing. The healer should practice yoga and Tai Chi, and fill himself with every possible form of positive healing energy. Filling up with energy can come from earth energy, heavenly energy, and so on.

It is important that at the end of every treatment, there is an electrical grounding from the healer's hands (using the "rooting" technique, in which one visualizes energy flowing into the earth) by touching a wall, or shaking and swinging the hands (preferably not onto any person or animal). The healer must see that there is a total separation between his energy and the patient's aura, and must "empty himself" in his imagination of the patient's condition of disease. Every now and then, it is a good idea for the healer to be treated by another healer, as well as draw energy from natural surroundings.

9. The aura

The aura and the energy centers (chakras) constitute the principal spiritual energy field for healing, and for that reason, they will be dealt with in separate chapters.

The aura is the manifestation of our electro-magnetic field. It is the sum total of the radiation that we emit. The aura appears around the body. It is influenced by fixed factors: food, heredity, the accumulation of previous memories, and so on, as well as variable factors: environmental conditions, conditions of life, levels of development, and so on.

The aura is our most holistic expression. It expresses all the strata of the body, the spirit, and the soul. This means that it is the healing field according to which the healer diagnoses the disease and cures it - possibly a long time before the symptoms occur. The aura is a collection of information about various processes, and of hereditary and environmental imbalances in the entire person. The aura, which is colored and has electro-magnetic manifestations, is a means by which it is possible to locate diseases of the delicate bodies that constitute the life force. It is composed of many layers within one another, like onion skins, and is linked to the energy centers (chakras) and from there to the rest of the body via plexuses to the nervous systems, the glands and the internal secretory system.

The aura manifests every illness and state of health.

It is radiated from inanimate objects, plants, and animals. The aura is the delicate expanse between the life force - universal energy - and the person. This occurs mainly through one of the layers, which is called the ethereal layer, through which the healer cures. The aura can be photographed by a special photographic technique, and according to various factors that are visible in it, it is possible to locate diseases. It transpires that a long time before the appearance of the symptoms of the disease, its presence is already identifiable in the aura, and for this reason, healing therapy is preventive therapy.

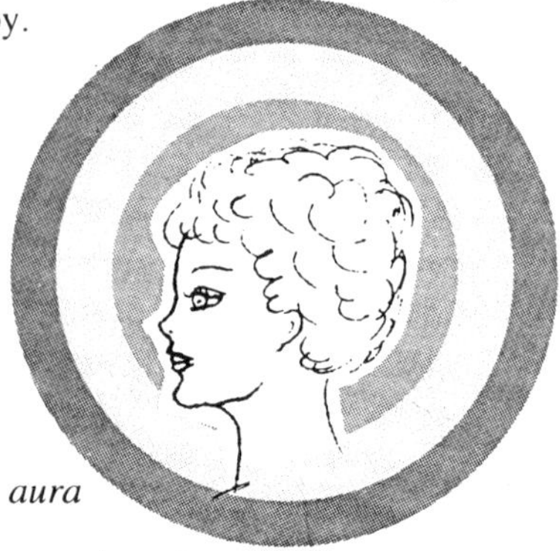

The various layers of the aura

It has been found that the aura is recharged every now and then, and the manifestation of its color comes from electrical currents, from vibrations, and from various influences. The basis for it starts during pregnancy, and it is more or less constant, but with the development of consciousness and awareness, it changes, mainly as a result of lifestyle, nutrition, diseases, health, the influences of ecological and environmental tensions, interpersonal relationships, past and present memories, negative or positive thoughts, music, colors, sport, crystals, and other factors, including medications, alcohol, drugs, plant essences, energetic atmosphere, surroundings, the company of people, mood, love, sex, enjoyment, calmness, meditation.

Historical Survey

We have evidence from the dawn of history that the aura can be seen. In his book, "The Third Eye," the Tibetan monk, *L. Rampa,* describes the moment he began to see auras. There are testimonies to seeing the auras of Buddha and Jesus. In Judaism, too, the ray of light that shone out of Moses' face when he came down from Mt. Sinai is mentioned. If this is the case, it seems that the auras of holy people or spiritual leaders are manifested more powerfully. In the drawings of various ancient cultures, the Aztecs and the Mayans, the aura appears. With the ancient Egyptians, we can find hats, which were apparently an expression of the electrical structure in their auras. Christian paintings show the auras of saints in different ways. The Ba'al Shem Tov tells about "a man from whose head pure light emanates until the heavens." The aura is the personal manifestation of the energy field of human beings, of inanimate objects, of plants or of animals.

Already in the 11th century (1020), attempts were made to describe the ethereal layer as the fourth state of matter after solid, liquid, and gas. The research on this topic received scientific impetus only at the end of the 19th century and the beginning of the 20th century (see chart in chapter 4). Already then, and following the theories of Pythagoras, Paracelsus, and Mesmer, it was understood that it was a question of an electro-magnetic field - the whole expression of energy.

The first photograph was taken at the end of the 19th century, and there tiny lines shining from a person's hand can be seen by clairvoyants. In 1908, Dr. Kilner began to take an interest in the aura as a result of theosophical writings that he had read on the topic of "The Aura and the Invisible Power of Vitality." Dr. Kilner was head of a department at St. Thomas' Hospital in London, which specialized in healing with electric shocks. He discovered that with practice, everyone can see the aura and distinguish its layers. In 1908, he attempted to cover a sheet of glass with a substance called dicyanin, and began to train his eyes to see complementary colors, in preparation for seeing the aura. He claimed that the aura was a diagnostic tool of the first order. By means of it, it is possible to predict diseases and preempt them. In 1911, he published research and diagrams in his book "The Human Aura," and produced eyeglasses for seeing the aura. According to his observations, there are differences between the auras of men and those of women, children, and pre-pubescent girls. It is possible to identify the auras of various diseases (such as hysteria, epilepsy, and insanity) or of pregnancy. Research that was performed subsequently by Dr. Piercus in the USA corroborated Kilner's findings. *Piercus* discovered that, if a good diagnosis is performed, it is indeed possible to discover signs of a disease that have not yet manifested themselves in the physical body.

In the 1920s and 1930s, a Russian scientist by the name of Igorevitch discovered that every living cell produces invisible radiation. He also noticed that a cell culture is enhanced and made healthy by healing and quartz crystal radiation.

After World War II, the first aura photograph was taken by the Russian researcher and technician, Simian Kirlian, who was involved in the technical side of medical equipment. He noticed that when a patient was linked to a machine that operated on very high-frequency electricity, an electrical spark or an electrical discharge occurred - a flash with a unique character - around the area of the photograph's contact. Following this, he constructed an instrument by means of which he photographed objects surrounded by a shining and glowing aura, using regular photographic film. "Kirlian photography" is named after him.

A Russian botanist brought him two leaves that had been picked at the same time to examine. The leaves looked identical and healthy, but in the photograph, one of them appeared weak with faded colors. Kirlian apologized for the failure of the experiment, but the botanist explained that the leaf with the weak aura had been taken from a sick plant. Kirlian photographed an incomplete leaf, and to his great surprise, its aura remained whole. This explains the "phantom" phenomenon experienced by amputees, as if the amputated limb or organ is still there. The body has a whole, clear, basic aura, which is the ethereal layer of the aura. Kirlian photography corroborated ancient knowledge about concealed energy currents and their connection to internal organs.

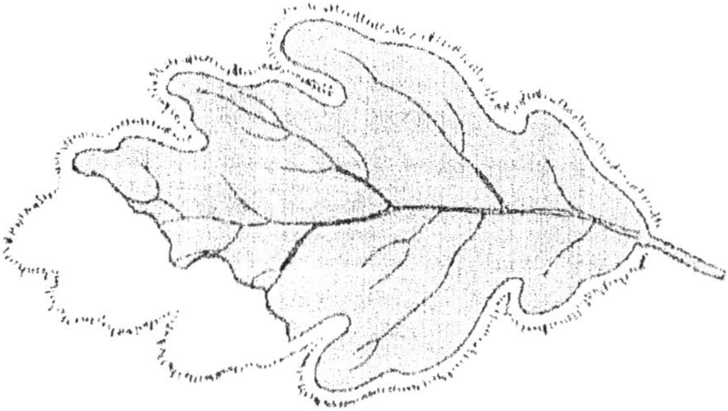

Torn leaf still has complete aura.

The layers of the aura

The aura consists of several layers. Each layer has its own vibration, and therefore stores different information. There are several ways to divide up the different layers, and several ways to relate to them.

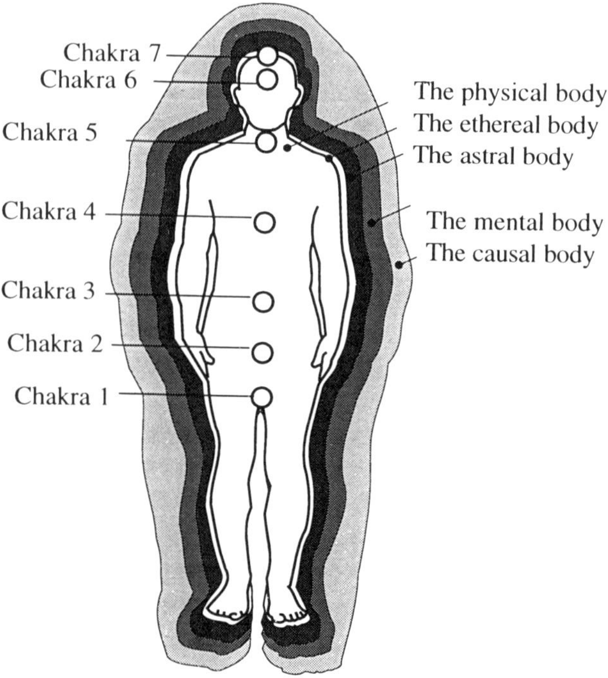

Theosophical division: Theosophy, meaning "divine wisdom," was a spiritual movement from the 19th century, which supported, among other things, the idea that there were seven interrelated elements in the aura. Alongside the physical body, there are also the ethereal, astral, mental, causal, and other bodies.

The ethereal body: This is a stage between substance and energy. This is the layer that is closest to the physical body (at a distance of about two inches). In a special photograph of the aura, this layer is seen as a white-bluish light that envelops the body. It constitutes a kind of double for the body, which is why amputees feel a reaction or pain in the amputated limb or organ, since the latter continues to manifest itself in an ethereal manner (a fact that has been proved in Kirlian and other photographs of the aura). The function of this high-energy layer is to revitalize the body's energy and recharge it, and mainly to join the universal life energy to the physical body. This life force - the Prana - is drawn in via breathing-air-sun, and from there spreads all over the body. Healers with extrasensory vision see this body as a weave of clear, thin lines (called nadis) that look like junctions of energy of an nervous electrical current. In a sick person, they look limp, and in a healthy person, they are strong and clear. This life force is sensitive to internal and external influences.

The ethereal body is nourished by sun, air, light, and light color, and it is damaged by smoke, alcohol, drugs, and an unhealthy lifestyle, and for that reason, it changes.

The astral body: This contains the chakras that are connected to it. It has a thin, separating boundary line, but also connects it to the ethereal and physical bodies. The astral body is located at a distance of about four inches from the physical body. This layer contains sensations and feelings - the intuitive ones - and is released during sleep by means of colors. It can be treated and balanced by every method of holistic healing, especially those tht focus on vibrations. It is possible to influence it using vibrational healing methods.

Many diseases originate from an imbalance in this layer. An "astral trip" is a breach of the border with the ethereal layer, and is expressed in dreams. Every kind of extreme behavior is an expression of emotional imbalance. In people who are ruled by their emotions, such as anger, guilt, and so on, this layer is not balanced. These people allow themselves to be drawn to negative energies that cause diseases.

The mental body: This body is made up of thoughts. Thought is a delicate, invisible substance that has form, color, and its own vibration. Every thought creates a morphological template that has energy. Thoughts have a great deal of power, and if thought is directed with strong and constant will power, it can change things - destroy or build them. Thoughts create diseases or build health, and they should therefore be treated very seriously. The most effective therapy for them is healing using a mental approach (see mental healing).

The causal body: This is the body that preserves the essence of the person's previous memories: knowledge, moral lessons, and experience that we have accumulated in the past (knowledge that is concealed in our brain), and it is capable of expressing the reasons for the spiritual vocation of every person.

Division according to P.B. Brennan

According to *Brennan*'s division, each layer in the aura is linked to a chakra, and its manifestation in the front of the body is different than at the back. In the front, the emotional centers are found, and at the back, the will centers.

Physical body:		
Layer I:	The ethereal body	Linked to the sex chakra and physical pleasures.
Layer II:	The emotional body	Linked to the emotional chakra.
Layer III:	The mental body	Linked to thought.
Emotional body:		
	The astral body	Linked to the heart chakra.
Spiritual body:		
	The ethereal-physical body	Linked to the chakras of expression, speech, listening, and will.
	The "divine"-emotional body	Linked to the universal love chakra.
	The "temple"-mental body	Linked to our highest spiritual chakra.

Division according to Austrum_

In his book, "Aura," the researcher Austrum points out that the aura is divided into the following parts: the aura of health (containing the ethereal, physical, and energetic aura), the vital body of the aura, the cognitive plane, the astral body of the aura, the mental body of the aura (lower and upper), and the spiritual body of the aura (the highest).

Every aura body, layer or stratum, has a different thickness, ranging from a fraction of an inch to a couple of inches. The diameter of a normal aura is generally as wide as the outstretched arms.

An additional division identifies three levels in the aura: the skeleton (bones); the flesh (blood), and the nerves. Each one involves a different diagnostic and therapeutic method of healing.

Connection between the aura, the chakras, and human wholeness

According to various theories, the ethereal body constitutes a field for filtering and transferring the link between human wholeness (subtle bodies) and the universal life energy. Via openings, or power stations, there are energy intersections that are called "chakras." There are systems of node-like intersections (the binding of nerve endings and the channeling and conveying of energy) and meridians, which are delicate energy conveyors (similar to blood flowing in blood vessels) to the internal secretory glands, and linked to every cell in the body. These energy openings filter the Chi energy, concentrate it, and distribute it below the skin, through the ethereal body. When the healer administers treatment, he balances the energy through these openings by radiating healing energy through them.

The manifestations of illnesses in the aura

In the UK and the USA, this subject began to be investigated only in the 60s, mainly with the publication of secret research. Gradually, it became known that a disease can manifest itself in different forms, such as: a "hole" in the aura, "lines," various marks such as spots, stripes or kinds of protrusions, dirt, or faded color, changing colors, and compression. Kirlian photography was perfected, and the radionic field helped in this. B. Brennan discovered in her observations that fear, anger, fatigue, sleeplessness, sadness, hatred, and so on, accumulate, and manifest themselves in the aura. She identified places of diseases, and described them as "frozen," "stuck," "shrunken," "tight," "outward-escaping," or "dirty" energy on the aura field (phlegm, mucus). The disease manifests itself in "defense mechanisms," and the person tries to survive at any price. Every such defense mechanism creates information in the aura layer. The color of the aura as well as its shape - compression, brightness, its appearance from the right or the left of the person, and other factors - all contribute to the information.

The mutual influence of relationships: anger, power struggles, nervousness, hysteria - all change the color of the aura, as do injuries, traumas and various situations of stress. The aura can become weak as a result of many deliberations and doubts, an unhealthy lifestyle, and a lack of physical and energetic charging.

Children see auras, and they tend to reveal this in their drawings or in their games in various ways; however, when adults (who no longer see auras) challenge their testimonies, they "stop" seeing them. According to B. Brennan, when a person gives free rein to a subject that he loves or which gives him a feeling of well-being, this is expressed in his aura. In the same way, medications and drugs have an effect. According to Brennan's observations, every tumor - benign or malignant - is revealed as a dark cloud in the vulnerable area and as a cut in the area that has lost its balance. Any deterioration in the situation will first be seen in the aura. Stressful situations, which can derive from internal or external problems, are manifested in the aura. The aura acts as a kind of delicate, colored seismograph to locate them.

The aura's signals are mainly via the colors. The interpretation of the colors and the changes are still being disputed. Some of the interpretations are presented below.

The dominant color in the aura and its significance

Cold colors: introversion, coldness, spirituality
Warm colors: creativity, extroversion, vitality
White: Extremely lofty color, in which all the colors are combined. Indicates light, purity, self-control, reaching enlightenment, spiritual development, and love or vanity.
Black: The need for self-concentration, the need to be in the center.
Pink: Universal love, art, beauty, desire for security or pampering, sensitivity, femininity, softness, emotion, etc.
Yellow: Representing the intellect from slyness (mustard yellow) to shyness (orange yellow); deep yellow: emphasis on the ego; light yellow: charisma and self-confidence.
Orange: Vitality, joy, energy; when impaired: stomach, spleen, pancreas, kidney problems - especially if the color is muddy (a lack of calcium, and so on).
Red: Anger, selfishness, impulsive and hot-tempered nature, passion, lust, vitality, activity, materialism, compulsive behavior (deep red).
Purple: Spirituality, healing; a muddy color tells of allergies and skin problems; deep purple: occasional exhaustion because of intensity; light purple: spirituality, intuition.
Green: Growth, feeling of change; a muddy color indicates problems in the tissues, heart, head, and intestines.

Blue: Inner information, intuition, healing, spiritual calm, wisdom, coldness, introversion.

10. Energy centers (chakras)

Chakra ("wheels" in Sanskrit) are generators, "power stations" that create energies. They are kind of whirlpools of energy, which are linked physically to the brain and to both sides of the spinal column, to the hormonal glands, and to the nerve ganglions. Their purpose is to pick up the energy and channel it, to absorb vital energy from the universe and distribute it evenly throughout the body. The chakras are linked to the rest of the parts of the body, and focus awareness and the various influences of the aura. The aim of healing is to balance their energies. Everyone has chakras, some of which are open, and others closed. Their imbalance causes illness. These key points store information about the entire body, and each one of them is linked to a layer in the aura. There are about 50 chakras in the body, of which seven are of cardinal importance. The small chakras are present in representative body parts, such as the palm of the hand and the sole of the foot. They are used to examine the wholeness of the person. The chakras behave in accordance with the principles of polarity, and changes along their axes are manifested in the colors of the aura. In the opinion of P. Randall, breathing, yoga and meditation are all ways of cleansing and charging the chakras. The healer draws universal energy from the air and exhales into the chakras at a rate that is appropriate to the person, and the vibration balances the energy. It is possible to cleanse and purify the chakras by means of crystals, colors, and sounds. Bach Flower Remedies can also be adapted to treating chakra problems.

The chakra can be examined by means of the pendulum. According to Brennan, if it is blocked or locked, the pendulum will indicate this fact by means of a counterclockwise motion. The chakra can also be activated by visualization, colors, crystals, sounds, movements, yoga, Tai Chi, and so on.

Chakra I: The Base Chakra

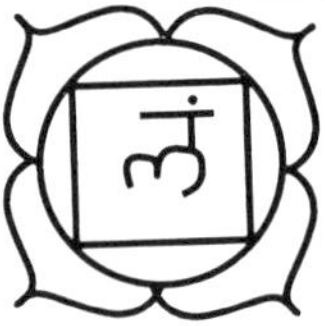

Muladhara in Sanskrit
Number: 1
Element: Earth
Color: Red
Sound: A (do) - Lam
Mantra: Lang
Location: Coccyx, between the anus and the genitals
Gland: Adrenal, connected to the sympathetic nervous system, to withstanding situations of anxiety, to survival
Nerve plexus: Tail plexus, at the end of the spinal column
Sense: Smell (earth)
Planet: Mars
Organs: Lower spinal column, anus, rectum, lower digestive system, outer genitals (penis, vagina), lower pelvis, legs, soles of feet, knees, blood circulation, blood pressure, nails, teeth.
When in balance: A great deal of physical strength, power, vitality, survival (fighting or escape mechanism), adaptability to reality and frameworks, endurance, ability to change, grounding, sense of orientation, ability to inspire belief, sensuality, love and enjoyment of sexual intercourse, not suspicious, affectionate, desire and lust for life.

Situation of excess: *Physical* (diseases): high blood pressure, temperature, flatulence, lower back, bleeding hemorrhoids, anus, recurring vaginal and urinary tract infections, foot and knee pains, edema, sore, protruding veins, leg pains, kidney stones, nervousness, sexual arousal, infections, hyperactivity. *Emotional*: Addiction to money, materialism, fanatic and extreme frameworks, escaping into work and become addicted to it, difficulty in adapting to changes and new frameworks, physical and mental domination, indiscriminate and compulsive sexual lust.

Situation of lack: *Physical* (diseases): anemia, poor blood circulation, low blood pressure, general feeling of coldness, cold, weak feet, frequent falls, impotence, leg and lower pelvic fractures, sexual frigidity, prolapsed rectum and anus, lack of physical strength, fainting spells. *Emotional*: feeling of not being loved, of not being popular, of loneliness, of being neglected and abandoned, of insecurity, of instability; fear of falling and of being abandoned, paranoia, suspicion, lack of self-esteem, self-destruction, potential suicide, shame, lack of motivation to live, easily influenced, sensitive.

Treatment:

Exercise and yoga

Breathing: Inhale, pause after exhaling.

Calming the spinal column physically and in the imagination.

Bach Flower Remedies: cherry, clematis, pine, sweet chestnut.

Healing stones and crystals: smoky quartz, black obsidian, black onyx, red garnet, ruby, red jasper, bloodstone, hawk-eye, hematite

Chakra II: The Sacral (Sex) Chakra

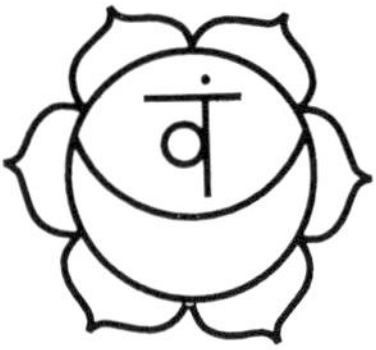

Savadhisthana in Sanskrit
Number: 2
Element: Water
Color: Orange
Sound: O (re) - Vam
Mantra: Yang
Location: Below the navel, the hollow of the groin, the pubis
Bone: The sacrum
Gland: Sex glands: ovary, testis, gonads
Nerve plexus: Parasympathetic plexus
Sense: Taste
Planet: Moon

Organs: Ovaries, testes, uterus, fallopian tubes, epididymis, sex hormones, lactiferous glands, skin, lower digestive system, bladder, lower back.

When in balance: No problems in sexual intercourse, in interpersonal relationships, or in communication; normal pregnancies and births, the ability to belong, creativity, identification with other people (but not to the point of being swallowed up), caring, friendly, a sense of humor, emotional strength, enjoyment of sex, and using it for personal release.

Situation of excess: *Physical* (diseases): lumbago (problematic lower back), slipped disk, uterine myoma, ovarian cysts, problems with sperm (quality and quantity), muscle spasms in the buttocks, problematic pelvis, difficulties in pregnancy and birth, urinary tract problems, edema, arthritis, excessive weight gain (difficulty in excreting undigested matter, takes in more than it excretes), need for frequent sex. *Emotional:* Lack of sex, exploiting people as sex objects, addictive, over-ambitious, over-identification, aggressive, manipulative, mistaken illusions.

Situation of lack: *Physical* (diseases): Amenorrhea or insufficient menstrual bleeding, weak and prolapsed uterus, problems of weakness in the genitals, defective sperm, weakness in the back, prolapsed bladder, lack of sexual stamina, lack of libido, frigidity, miscarriages, sterility, lack of milk in nursing mothers, muscle cramps and spasms, sensitivity to the surroundings and allergies. *Emotional:* Guilt feelings about sex and birth, a feeling of being exploited, humiliation, inhibitions, clinging without letting go, sexual repression, paralyzed by fear, excessive shyness, excessive sensitivity and vulnerability in interpersonal relations, concealing feelings, feeling of discontent toward oneself.

Treatment:

Submission and release of whatever is not digested (visualizations and positive thoughts)

Exercise and yoga.

Breathing: Pause after exhaling

Bach Flower Remedies: Crab apple, elm, oak, verbena, rock water

Crystals and stones: ruby, carnelian, orange agate, red sapphire

Chakra III: The Solar Plexus Chakra

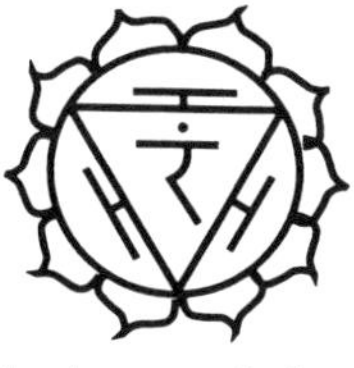

Manipura in Sanskrit
Number: 3
Element: Fire
Color: Yellow
Sense: Sight
Sound: M (mi) - Ram
Mantra: Rang
Location: From the belly to the diaphragm, below the sternum, diaphragm, stomach.

Gland: Pancreas, secretion of digestive juices and insulin for metabolism and the regulation of sugars.

Nerve plexus: The sympathetic nervous system inside the autonomic nervous system.

Planet: Sun, the source of the link between the astral and ethereal bodies

Organs: Diaphragm, stomach, duodenum, spleen, liver, gall bladder, small and large intestines, pancreas and the whole digestive system, middle back.

When in balance: Normal digestion, *joie de vivre*, self-respect, no need to be right all the time, not power-hungry or domineering, but assertive and standing up for oneself, knowing what one's uniqueness and strengths are without the need to prove it, spontaneity, self-confidence, will power, normal family relationships, enjoyment of good food, caring about spouse and children, showing uninhibited affection and emotion, comfortable, good powers of expression.

Situation of excess: *Physical* (diseases): Digestive problems: constipation, diarrhea, ulcer, stomach-aches, worms, Candida, heartburn, inflammation of the small and large intestines, flatulence, diabetes, hiatus hernia, cancer, intestinal tumors, gall stones, liver problems, digestive difficulties. *Emotional:* Negative and aggressive approach toward others and oneself, domineering, always wanting to be right, power-hungry, judgmental, perfectionist, excelling, compulsive, wanting to make an impression, rational without emotion, dependent, irascible, strong ego, addicted to work and personal justice, excessively rational, demanding, loathing authority or worshipping authority, complaining incessantly about the relationship, and placing one's partner in an eternal test situation.

Situation of lack: *Physical*: Poor digestion, lack of acidity and digestive strength to break down and absorb the food, poor intestinal movement, a paunch, allergy to food, lack of energy, prolapsed digestive organs, kidney insufficiency, weak blood flow in the abdomen, intestinal spasms, nausea. *Emotional:* Constant need for ego reinforcement, worry about one's image, blocked anger, fears, jealousy, guilt, greed for money, introversion, sentimentality, conscience that is not clear, indecisiveness, frustration following never-ending conflicts, confusion, negative attitude toward the surroundings, sleeplessness.

Treatment:

Control of the lust for power by means of visualizations and positive thoughts

Breathing: No pause between exhaling and inhaling

Exercise and yoga

Bach Flower Remedies: Aspen, birch, star of Bethlehem

Crystals and therapeutic stones: citrine, yellow topaz, rutile, tiger's-eye, yellow fluorite, malachite, cat's-eye

Chakra IV: The Heart Chakra

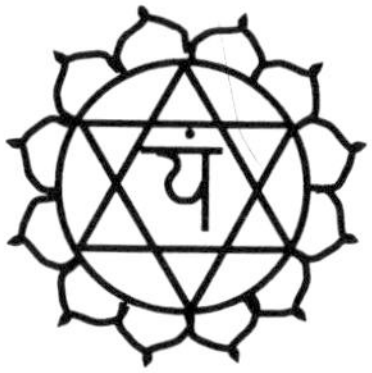

Anahata in Sanskrit

Number: 4

Element: Air

Color: Green

Characteristic: Unconditional acceptance of others

Sound: Ee (fa) - Yam

Mantra: Yang

Sense: Touch

Location: Between the nipples, middle back/chest vertebra

Gland: Thymus - immune system gland

Nerve plexus: The heart plexus

Planet: Venus

Organs: Heart, lungs, respiratory organs, bronchial tubes, trachea, esophagus, sternum, lymph and the immune system, breast, thymus, upper back, shoulder muscle

When in balance: Unconditional love that expects nothing in return, humane, considerate, serene, balanced, healing ability, compassionate, supportive of every person, friendly, aspiring to give and help, and also knowing how to receive, in good contact with one's emotions, strong will power, waiting for the suitable partner, not compromising, adapting to the state of being a couple well, and into other relationships.

Situation of excess: *Physical* (diseases): Pneumonia, heart and circulatory problems, angina pectoris, coughing, tracheal problems, nausea, vomiting, stiff upper back muscles, shoulder blades, shoulders, clavicle, cramps and pains, frozen shoulder, increased heart rate, problems in upper limbs, heart pains, heart attacks, respiratory difficulties, asthma, hypertension, lung cancer. *Emotional:* Demanding, shouldering everyone else's burdens, not relying on others, burdening others, critical, wanting love at any price and at any terms, problems of giving and taking, controlling others, moodiness, difficulty in reaching decisions, over-ambitious, tense, angry, feeling unworthy of love, negative attitude toward people, overly critical, acquisitive, melodramatic, moody, conditional love.

Situation of lack: *Physical:* Lack of blood, weak lungs, fatigue, exhaustion, smoking, impaired immunity, allergy, weak heart, emphysema, weakness in the diaphragm, weakness in the blood. *Emotional:*

Inability to ask others for help, fear of being rejected, unimpressive, or abandoned, frustrated, and weak, indecisive, hesitant, deliberating, difficulty in expressing emotion, fear of being free and happy, feeling of being unworthy of love and forgiveness, self-pitying.

Treatment:

Providing service, coping with remoteness, hatred, lack of quiet, visualization, positive thinking

Exercise: Yoga

Bach Flower Remedies: Centaury, chicory, honeysuckle, rock rose, red chestnut

Crystals: Rose quartz, rhodonite, green and pink tourmaline, emerald, jade, unicate.

Breathing: Breathing without pausing

Chakra V: The Throat Chakra

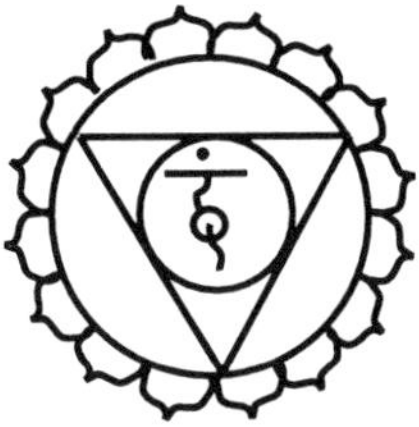

Vishuddha in Sanskrit

Number: 5

Field: Communication

Color: Blue

Sound: Oh (so)

Mantra: Hang

Location: Throat, neck, mouth, and neck vertebrae

Gland: Thyroid

Nerve plexus: Throat

Sense: Hearing

Planet: Mercury

Organs: Throat, thyroid gland, lobe of the thyroid gland, vocal cords, neck, tonsils, epiglottis, tongue, gums, teeth, palate, ears, and neck muscles

When in balance: Creative, ability to express oneself, enters a state of relaxation easily, trusting, communicative, without harsh judgment and criticism, self-awareness and self-identity concerning one's uniqueness, sense of timing and immediacy, receptive to spiritual learning, good connection between common sense and intuition, and between the conscious and the unconscious, open to change, flexible, connection between the new and the old, one's own master, accomplishes goals and objectives, understanding that one is the source of one's own life, patience.

Situation of excess: *Physical* (diseases): Chronic throat inflammations, expectorating, phlegm, excessive smoking, ears, stuttering, frequent colds, growths on the vocal cords, runny nose, hoarseness, gum and teeth problems, hyperthyroidism. *Emotional:* Conceited, not in tune with one's true needs, negative thinking and expression, rapid and indistinct speech, unclear relationships with others, inconsistent communication, not reliable, shirker, liar, schemer, violent.

Situation of lack: *Physical:* Hypothyroidism, depressions, irregularity of calcium and potassium, lack of strength in the neck, throat, shoulders, clavicle, weak muscles, slow, weak speech, loss of voice, weak voice. *Emotional:* Introverted, closed, frightened, shy, quiet, restrained, excessive fatigue, mental exhaustion, swallows insults, hesitates to speak, does not respond to opponents, obsequious, not reliable, secretive, vulnerable, often depressed.

Treatment:

Communication by means of visualization and positive thinking

Breathing: Pausing after exhaling

Crystals: Turquoise, aquamarine, chrysocolla, blue topaz

Exercises and yoga

Bach Flower Remedies: agrimony, mustard, oats, willow.

Chakra VI: The Third Eye Chakra

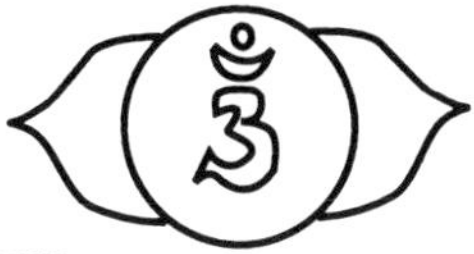

Ajna in Sanskrit
Number: 6
Element: Wind
Color: Indigo
Sound: Ohm (la) Ham Kisham
Sense: Intuition (extrasensory)
Mantra: Ohm (la) Kisham

Location: At the base of the skull, in the brain, on the forehead above and between the eyebrows

Gland: Hypophysis (the pituitary body of the brain)

Nerve plexus: The brain stem, senses, left eye

Organs: Sense organs, sight, auditory, olfactory, taste, endocrine system (supervision of the hormones), hypophysis, lower brain, left eye, ears

When in balance: Good imagination, creativity, positive thoughts, healthy senses, uniformity, flexibility in thought, wholeness of body, modest, spiritual, having access and a link to inner sources of knowledge, open to spiritual experiences, hormonal and immunity balance, telepathy, trusts oneself and superior forces, operates within freedom of thought, one's own master, unconcerned with glory, fame, ability to receive spiritual guidance, not afraid of death.

Situation of excess: *Physical* (diseases): Headache (forehead), communication problems in the senses: sight, hearing nose, ear, smell and taste, tinnitus, sinusitis, facial nerves, problems of sleep, concentration, perception, memory, imagination. *Emotional:* Mental diseases, negative thinking, pride, detachment from reality, alienated from the surroundings, impaired senses, strong ego, refusal to communicate with the surroundings, dogmatic, boastful, power-hungry.

Situation of lack: Weak vision, senses, confusion, nervous weakness of the face, headaches, bruises and problems with the skin of the face, baldness, dandruff. *Emotional:* Depression, sadness, lack of assertiveness, over-sensitivity toward others, withdrawn, mental and spiritual exhaustion, fear of success, undisciplined.

Treatment:

Intuition and open thought (visualizations, commitment)

Crystals and stones: Sodalite, chlorite, amethyst, lapis lazuli, calcite, quartz

Exercise and Yoga

Bach Flower Remedies: Beech, chestnut bud, willow, olive, vine, white chestnut

Breathing: Pausing after exhaling

Chakra VII: The Crown Chakra

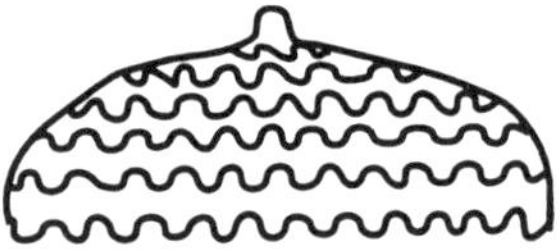

Sahasrara in Sanskrit

Number: 7

Element: Light, ether

Color: White (an absence of color, just light), purplish

Sound: No sound (or Ti)

Sense: Intuition (extrasensory)

Mantra: Ohm

Location: At the top of the skull, on most of the area of the head

Gland: Pineal

Nerve plexus: Central (cerebral) nervous system

Organs: Brains, central nervous system, sensory-motor actions, thought, upper brain, right eye

Planet: Neptune

When in balance: Has cosmic spiritual

awareness, operates according to intuitive ability, obeys inner voices, sees and hears invisible things, but also grounded and practical, can explain himself, does not make mistakes, linked to moral cosmic knowledge, modest, does only what is right for his development without harming anyone, is married to the partner that suits him, lives in the surroundings that are appropriate to him.

Situation of excess: *Physical* (diseases): Headaches, chronic migraines, scabies, skin diseases, scalp infections, problems with concentration and memory, Alzheimer. *Emotional:* Confusion, spaced-out, autism, paranoia, senility, sleep and nervous disturbances.

Situation of lack: Mental and spiritual fatigue, exhaustion, epilepsy, lack of orientation, vertigo, xxxx, baldness, hair loss, dizziness, lack of memory, loss of balance, sleeplessness. *Emotional:* Fantasizes, not grounded, prone to delusions, not practical, speaks out of context, not realistic, does not do things that suit his uniqueness, demented to the very edge of sanity.

Treatment:

Self-unity (visualization, positive thought)

Breathing: Stopping after exhaling

Exercise and yoga

Bach Flower Remedies

Crystals and stones: Quartz, crystal, opal, diamond, moonstone.

According to various theories, an additional important chakra should be added to the seven main chakras. It is located between the base chakra and the sacral chakra. The eighth chakra is the spleen chakra, which, according to other theories, is the second chakra.

The spleen is the center of the astral enlightenment system. The vital body, which picks up Chi (Prana) from the sun, absorbs vitality from the atmosphere and distributes it to the seven colors of the spectrum, and from there to the various body parts, in this way nourishing the nervous system. This is the chakra, or "sub-chakra," that helps when the base chakra is weakened. It contains the same number of colors as the spectrum. Healers are nourished by this chakra. If this energy is lacking in the nervous system, the person becomes sensitive and very stimulated. Spending time in natural surroundings, especially beside pine and eucalyptus trees, makes this chakra healthy. When a person is healthy and full of this chakra, he is liable to be "pumped" by a sick person, who "sucks" the energy out of him via the chakra.

11. Treatment Techniques in Healing

Treatments

According to Reiki healing: The treatments are performed after diagnosis (scanning), which is done by placing the hands in various positions on the body, and with the help of various symbols. The different positions begin from the head (the crown), and move to the eyes, the ears, the temples, the back of the head, the nape, the clavicle (the heart), the spleen, the liver (below the chest), the abdomen (around the navel), the groin, the region where the legs join. In addition, the hands are placed on the palms, on the knees, and on the feet, and also on the back.

This treatment is performed after studying and attunement (preparations, protections, charging of the healer). A person can treat himself or others. He holds his hands in each position for 3-5 minutes, and eventually finds himself at peace.

In Reiki, there is specialized treatment of different types of diseases, such as arthritis, heart problems, gynecological problems, headaches, back problems, and so on. Every disease has a suitable hand position that is meant specifically for it.

According to B. Brennan: B. Brennan has been involved in research and healing for many years. She believes, as do many others, that treatment must begin with the preparation of the healer, and after that comes the cleansing of the aura of energetic waste. The cleansing expels, drains, and concentrates the waste that blocks the aura and accompanies good energy. The way to do this, in her opinion, is, among others, from bottom to top, or by shaking the hands in a certain way. After cleansing the spinal column, cleansing is done in certain places that are blocked and inhibit the flow of the aura, examination and cleansing of the chakras, and the rebuilding of the energy flow. This is done by means of placing the hands on the chakras and adjusting the healer's energy systems to those of the patient.

According to Weinman: According to Weinman, it is possible to organize energetic balance by means of equalizing the energy between pairs of chakras. Moreover, the healer must recharge himself by inhaling higher energy: "earth" energy, "sun" energy, colors, visualizations, and other techniques.

Cleansing the aura

According to various theories, cleansing the aura is the central and most important treatment. It is performed at three levels: "bones," "blood," and "nerves." The healer passes his hands over the body or at a short distance from it. It is possible to cleanse each level separately using the following technique:

The bone level: In straight lines along the lines of the skeleton, close to the body and at a distance from it.

The blood level: In circular lines to symbolize the cyclical nature of blood.

The nerve level: By moving the fingers and administering light pinches like a nervous tremor.

It is possible to cleanse by moving the hand down the body in a line, "collecting" the waste, and shaking off one's hands to discard negative energies.

It is possible to get rid of energetic waste by means of a quartz crystal and healing stones, especially by placing it in the opposite direction to the body.

Healing techniques

It is possible to hold the hands in different ways above the aura: flat, in a pyramidal shape, making them tremble, pinching, emphasizing one of the fingers, using the back of the hands, using the hands as a kind of magnet, waving them, cleansing, and so on. Sometimes currents are felt, and then the healer must distinguish whether his hand absorbed or transmitted energy. According to the reactions of the patient and the sensations of the healer with the help of a pendulum and additional means, it is possible to examine the results of the treatment.

During the treatment, the healer imagines the patient becoming healthy, or the diseased organ becoming balanced. He imagines that a healing color emanates from his hands, and prays for the recovery of the patient. He can be in a meditative state of alpha waves, and then the treatment is more intense.

Every disease has several healing techniques. Treatment that is administered for the first time has a special technique, and it belongs to the field of giving first aid.

12. Healing exercises for self-development

Healing can be developed, perfected, and made more effective with exercises. A person can improve his healing ability both for himself and for others. Every exercise should be related to with a great deal of responsibility. Remember that healing can bring about a great improvement, especially by means of spiritual development, and not only in a technical manner.

Exercises for self-healing

Close your eyes, sit calmly, inhale and fill your lungs, and exhale slowly, several times. Relax every part of your body physically and in your imagination. Concentrate mainly on your fingers, feel that they are warm and heavy, and try to create a feeling of light around every finger in your imagination. Imagine that sick parts of the body (cramps, pains) are receiving light from your fingers. In your imagination, breathe into and out of the diseased organ, and imagine that the area is illuminated and made healthy.

Sit calmly, close your eyes, and let your body rest. Breathe gently. Exhale and inhale slowly. Relax your body in your imagination, part after part. Direct your consciousness (concentrate your attention) toward the region of your fingers, and try to imagine them filled with light or warmth or any other sensation that was not there previously. Now create in your imagination a kind of "imaginary ball," and try to place it gently on the painful place for a few minutes. Follow and check if indeed there has been an improvement in the pain. It is also possible to imagine that the pain is being "drawn" out; shake your hands in order to neutralize the negative energies.

Exercises for seeing and feeling the aura

Feeling the aura between the fingers

* Place the fingers next to one another, to see and feel a kind of layer of light, heat, color, or magnetic attraction between them. Move the hands away from each other and bring them closer, and pay attention to what you feel. You must notice that even when you stretch out your hands, there are kind of lines or threads of energy that remain joined.

* The hands are used as antennas for absorbing and giving out energy. The nerves branch out in them, and the meridians begin and end. The hands charge energy and also radiate it. It is possible to use them to see an aura.

For seeing the aura

* Focus energy in the spread hand, so that the thumb is at a distance from the rest of the fingers. Make a kind of window and look through it at a white wall. Alternately shut your eyes and open them, and look at the white wall.

* Look at a person, and try to check on a white background if you can see any color next to his body.

* At the beginning, it is possible to use glasses in order to see the aura, but the eye must be trained to see complementary colors. For instance, look at the color green, close your eyes, and look at a white wall, and see its complementary color - red (according to Newton's theory).

* Close your eyes, and try to feel, while closing your eyes, what the color of the aura is, after having gotten an impression of the person.

Feeling the aura on the patient's body

* Feeling the aura is easier to do. The body must be scanned from top to bottom with each hand separately, trying to feel (with eyes closed) if you can sense reactions (heat, cold, prickling).

* You should practice drawing the aura according to feeling.

Exercises for energetic recharging

* Work in pairs and try to see the positive details in your partner. Transmit to him positive feelings and ask what he feels.

* Feel "an imaginary filling-up with light" by means of inhaling, and visualize yourself being recharged from three sources: from an upper source, a kind of white sunbeam that enters a hole in the crown, fills the spinal column, and from there spreads all over the body; from an earth source (from the feet); from the heart.

Exercise for enlarging the aura and energetic protection

* With eyes closed, after inhaling and exhaling slowly, feel in your imagination that your spinal column, from the crown of your head to the tip of your coccyx, is painted in a luminous white color. Inhale and feel the light color entering, and exhale and feel the dark color leaving.

* In your imagination, feel that you are surrounded by a bubble of light; enlarge it by breathing, until you have the feeling that you are at the center of the light. Afterward, go back and reduce it to its normal state, and feel that you are "protected from negative influences."

* You can hold your hands on your solar plexus and breathe. This is an important energy center, the source

of strength and vitality. While breathing, feel that this center is filling up with light, and strengthening you.

Exercise for cleansing energetic "waste and protection"

Place your hands in the region of the navel, and imagine kind of pure water washing every part of the body, from the navel to every cell and organ. Feel results by exhaling.

Astrolog Publishing House
P. O. Box 1123, Hod Hasharon 45111, Israel
Tel: 972-9-7412044
Fax: 972-9-7442714
E-Mail: info@astrolog.co.il
Astrolog Web Site: www.astrolog.co.il

ISBN 965-494-100-7

Published by Astrolog Publishing House 2000

Printed in Israel
2 4 6 8 10 9 7 5 3 1